2012

NA

CreateSpace

Lung Cancer
Remedy-True Story
+ bonus
Story of Ike
Meshulam's twice
survival of lung
cancer using both
conventional and
natural means, plus
bonus remedy for
mucous building
diseases, such as CF

LUNG CANCER REMEDY- TRUE STORY +BONUS

A little bit of history- My husband Ike had a lung cancer in the

_____

lower right lobe of his lung in the year 2000. It appeared following a heart attack. One-fourth of the lower right lobe was removed (The cancer was about the size of a quarter)

with no
follow-up
treatment
required.

IN THE
SPRING OF
2008, MY
HUSBAND
had chest
pains and

_____

was
admitted to
the hospital
for an
angioplasty.
At that time,
by chance, a
new lung
cancer was
found in the
UPPER lobe
of his right
lung.
Starting the
end of March

or early
April of
2008, Ike
was referred
to a local
hospital for
radiation
treatments.
These were
administere
d weekly
over the next
8 weeks. The
surgeon was
unable to

remove the upper lobe of the right lung because, according to my husband, of the proximity to many blood vessels in the surrounding area. Also if it could be removed in its entirety, Ike would probably need an oxygen tank. Henceforth, just a wedge was removed. Consequently, the radiation treatments were given. The cancer

this time was
about the
size of a fifty-
cent piece
and was
located on
the edge of
the upper
right lung.

Radiation
was targeted
to this area

after
surgery.
Supposedly,
the radiation
helped, but it
burned the
area and
produced
much
scarring of
the lung. It
also could
have caused
bleeding.
After the

———————————

radiation blood tests were done and the cancer was then found not only in the lung but also in one or two lymph nodes and in the LIVER!! They called this type of cancer an "adenocarcin oma." It is a very dangerous type of cancer. The Dr. referred to it as the "dead mans cancer, " according to Ike.

_____

Chemothera
py was
started
shortly after
the blood
tests showed
that the lung
cancer had
spread.
There were 4
weekly
sessions.
Blood tests

were done
again and
the lymph
node(s) and
liver were
clear.
Cancer,
however was
still in the
lung.

My husband
went into

———————————

remission as shown by several CAT Scans and 4 PET Scans following the chemotherapy treatments. The cancer was still in the lung, but not spreading. However, it could have flared up at any time and killed him, so we felt that something needed to be tried, as it seemed that all options were exhausted by the doctors. If your case is similar, this story

could save
your lives.
No
guarantees!

Here is the
remedy that
my husband
Ike tried at
my
suggestion

while he was
in remission

This is very
important!!!
There are no
guarantees
and other
treatments
were taken.
It is also

_____

important to note that Ike did

not go through any kind of detoxificatio n program. I don't know if the treatment would be more effective if

one embarks
on such a
program in
addition to
it. This is
what
appears to
me to have
worked in
getting rid of
that deadly
lung cancer.
Judge for
yourself. I
make no

---

claims that it will work for you.

For a little over 1 month Ike consumed:

1 large glass (roughly 16 oz.) of FRESH

carrot juice (organic is best) per day. Just juice the carrots in a good juicer

6-8 cups of red clover tea (steeped in a teapot makes it a bit easier, because it is readily on hand- ceramic teapot good- We used one about a quart and a half capacity. If you don't have enough tea, or you have only a one quart pot, you can steep some

more bags,
or bulk tea
w/a tea ball
in boiling
water. Just
pour over
bags in
ceramic
teapot and
let steep.
The longer
you steep
(replace the
teapot top
and let

steep) the
stronger the
tea gets. I
steeped the
tea for about
15-20
minutes.
Sometimes I
would forget
to take the
bags out.
The tea
tastes
pleasant
though, I

think. I used about 4 or 5 tea bags per pot, but there should be directions on the box for making a pot at a time. You can also make it by the cup of course. Red clover tea is not very

expensive
and can be
bought in
just about
any health
food store.
FYI- My
husband
took this
remedy at
6'1" tall,
about
250lbs.

CAUTION: If you have lung cancer, and have had radiation treatments, you may experience bleeding after taking this remedy. My husband was spitting blood profusely

_____

after the
month of
consuming
these two
things. He
had to go to
the hospital
to receive
platelets.

BUT—
following
this, there
was no
evidence of

malignancies in the blood tests and have been none since. Ike has negative monthly results for malignancies to this day.

USE the REMEDY at

---

your OWN
RISK!

Here is MY
reasoning as
to why the
bleeding
from the
lung MIGHT
have
occurred. I
am NOT a
PHYSICIAN. I
am just the
average Jane

with an opinion.

Since there was much scarring to the lung as a result of the radiation treatments and red clover tea happens to be a muscle relaxant,

———————————

maybe a tear
in the tissue
was
produced
from
consuming a
large
amount.
Also, as an
aside, Ike is
of Ashkenazi
Jewish
ancestry and
was told by a
doctor that

they bleed more than many. (An extra bonus FYI for Ashkenazi Jewish people)

A reason why, in my opinion, this remedy could have worked for

---

my husband
is that he
was told,
according to
him, by the
doctor, that
the
particular
area of the
lung where
his deadly
cancer was
located acts
like a
sponge. It

could have
directly
absorbed the
tea and
carrot juice.
Supposedly,
red clover
tea is an
effective
blood
purifier and
fights cancer.
Carrot juice
is also
supposedly

quite
effective
against it. I
came up with
this remedy
after reading
a work by an
herbalist
born in the
early
twentieth
century and
who is
deceased for
many years,

named Jethro Kloss. I don't remember where I read that the red clover tea is a muscle relaxant, but believe me, I know that it is from personal experience. I took it after drinking some wine. I had forgotten what I had read about it and I thought I was going to go into a coma! But I was okay. DO NOT CONSUME ALCOHOL AT ALL WITH

RED CLOVER TEA!

BONUS tidbit of info— Carrot juice supposedly removes mucus very effectively. Henceforth,

_____

it does stand
to reason
that it would
be effective
with any
disease
which
involves
mucus
buildup in
the body, e.g.
Cystic
Fibrosis.
This I think I
read about in

a very old book, possibly published in the 1960's called (I hope I remember the title correctly) NATURAL HEALTH.

Again—No guarantees-I

_____

have no clue
how much
carrot juice
to consume
in a Cystic
Fibrosis case,
but it's food
and not man-
made
medication.
Carrots also
can be eaten,
I think. I
don't know
which is

better or if
it's the same
in
effectiveness
or not.

Note-Carrots
are sweet, so
if you are
diabetic, be
sure to
consult a
physician
before

consuming
them.

It would be a
good idea to
consult with
a physician
or a
professional
who KNOWS
about
adverse drug
interactions
with food
and herbs

before trying
anything
presented
here, and I
make no
claims that it
will cure
anyone of
anything, or
produce
desired
benefits. (My
writing
could be
better but

the content is there.

Information given concerning my husband's case was contributed from memory by my husband and me.

By:

**Cheryl
Rovira-
Meshulam**

_____

www.ingramcontent.com/pod-product-compliance
Lightning Source LLC
Chambersburg PA
CBHW062301290526
45794CB00006B/2656